Watch Your Weight New Complete Cookbook 2024: 20 Smart Points To Hit Your Weight Loss Goals in a Few Weeks, Delicious Recipes That Improve Overall Health & Make it an Effective Tool for Weight Loss

Clayton Thompson

Table of Contents

Chapter One

Navigating Dietary Preferences:

Creating inclusive dishes includes choosing diverse components. For a vegetarian variation, go for plant-based proteins like tofu or lentils. Replace dairy with plant-based alternatives for vegan choices. Choose gluten-free grains like quinoa to accommodate gluten-sensitive persons. Experimenting with varied tastes guarantees a rewarding experience for everyone.. Here's a thorough breakdown:

1. Vegetarian Options: Include a range of delectable and nutrient-rich meals that avoid meat but are still filled with proteins from plant-based sources such as beans, lentils, tofu, and quinoa.

2. Vegan Delights: Explore dishes that go beyond vegetarian by omitting all animal products, giving inventive and exciting plant-based alternatives for a full and balanced diet.

3. Gluten-Free Goodness: Recognize the requirements of people with gluten sensitivity or preferences, providing recipes that employ gluten-free grains like rice, quinoa, and gluten-free flour substitutes without sacrificing flavor or texture.

4. Low-Carb Creations: Address the popularity of low-carb diets by delivering dishes that are not only tasty but also conform to reduced carbohydrate content, integrating vegetables, lean meats, and healthy fats.

5. Flexitarian Flavors: Cater to the rising trend of flexitarianism, giving recipes that give flexibility in including occasional meat while largely concentrating on plant-based components.

6. Paleo Pleasures: Explore dishes matched with the Paleolithic diet, emphasizing natural foods, lean meats, fruits, and vegetables while avoiding processed foods, grains, and dairy.

7. Dairy-Free Delicacies: Acknowledge lactose intolerance or dairy-free preferences with recipes that employ alternative milk and cheese choices, ensuring that folks with dairy limitations may still enjoy delectable meals.

8. Nut-Free Nibbles: Recognize and handle nut allergies by providing dishes that avoid nuts but remain rich in flavor and nutritional value via substitute ingredients.

By presenting a range of recipes for varied dietary choices, this part guarantees that the "Watch Your Weight New Complete Cookbook 2024" becomes an inclusive resource, catering to the varying demands and interests of a wide audience.

Chapter Two

Superfoods Unveiled:

Consider mixing chia seeds into your morning yogurt or oatmeal for a fiber and omega-3 boost. Create a nutrient-packed smoothie by combining kale, blueberries, and a banana. Quinoa salads with a combination of bright greens make a pleasant and healthy dinner. These dishes may help with general health and assist weight control objectives. Here's a thorough breakdown:

1. Introduction to Superfoods: Begin by describing what superfoods are and emphasize their nutritional richness and health advantages. Superfoods are nutrient-rich foods thought to be extremely helpful for health and well-being.

2. Quinoa Power Bowls: Showcase quinoa as a superfood full of protein, fiber, and important elements. Provide recipes for vivid and fulfilling quinoa bowls, mixing them with a range of veggies, lean meats, and savory dressings.

3. Salmon Superstars: Feature salmon as a superfood strong in omega-3 fatty acids. Present dishes that emphasize the variety of salmon, from grilled filets to inventive salmon salads, stressing its contribution to heart health and weight control.

4. Blueberry Bliss: Highlight blueberries as antioxidant-rich superfoods. Include recipes for tasty blueberry-infused foods, such as smoothies, salads, and desserts, highlighting their potential advantages for weight management.

5. Kale Kick: Explore kale as a nutrient-dense leafy green. Provide ideas for kale-based salads, soups, and smoothies, stressing its high fiber and vitamin content to promote a balanced diet.

6. Avocado Elegance: Showcase avocados as a superfood rich in beneficial fats. Present ideas for avocado-centric meals, from guacamole to avocado toast, boosting fullness and taste in weight-conscious eating.

7. Chia Seed Marvels: Introduce chia seeds as a superfood rich in omega-3 fatty acids and fiber. Offer inventive ideas for chia seed puddings, smoothie bowls, and energy snacks, including their nutritional advantages.

8. Sweet Potato Supercharge: Feature sweet potatoes as a superfood rich in vitamins and fiber.

Provide ideas for savory and sweet foods, highlighting the flexibility of sweet potatoes in increasing satiety and supporting weight goals.

9. Turmeric Treasures: Explore turmeric as a superfood with anti-inflammatory qualities. Include recipes for turmeric-infused foods, such as golden milk and curries, emphasizing its possible health advantages.

10. Almond Alchemy: Highlight almonds as a superfood rich in healthy fats and minerals. Provide recipes for almond-based snacks, salads, and desserts, highlighting their potential role in a balanced diet.

By adding these superfoods into the cookbook, readers receive access to recipes that not only support their weight management objectives but also contribute to general well-being via the incorporation of nutrient-dense and health-promoting ingredients.

Chapter Three

Slow Cooker Wonders:

Utilize the slow cooker for nutritious meals by stocking it with lean meats like chicken or beans, along with a variety of veggies. Add aromatic herbs and spices for taste without unnecessary calories. The slow-cooking procedure enriches tastes while keeping your food nutrient-rich and supporting your weight-conscious aims. Here's a thorough breakdown:

1. Introduction to Slow Cooking: Begin by stressing the positives of using a slow cooker, such as convenience, time-saving, and the capacity to improve tastes via slow, gentle cooking.

2. Time-Saving Simplicity: Showcase dishes that need less preparation yet result in excellent and fulfilling dinners.

Slow cookers are perfect for busy persons seeking healthful solutions without lengthy hands-on cooking time.

3. Nutrient Preservation: Emphasize how slow cooking helps maintain the nutritional value of foods, ensuring that vitamins and minerals are kept in the final meals.

4. Lean Protein Creations: Feature dishes using lean protein sources, such as chicken, turkey, or plant-based proteins, cooked gently to increase softness and taste while making the meals ideal for weight-conscious aims.

5. Hearty Soups and Stews: Present recipes for hearty and nutritious soups and stews, showing the slow cooker's capacity to merge flavors and textures over time, resulting in soothing and full foods.

6. Vegetarian Slow Cooker Delights: Cater to vegetarians with dishes that center on slow-cooked veggies, legumes, and grains, giving plant-based alternatives that are both healthful and fulfilling.

7. Whole Grain Goodness: Explore the use of whole grains like quinoa, brown rice, and barley in slow cooker meals, boosting fiber-rich alternatives that promote weight control.

8. Versatile One-Pot Meals: Highlight the ease of one-pot meals in a slow cooker, reducing cleaning while increasing taste. Include dishes that mix protein, veggies, and grains in a single pot.

9. Infusing tastes with Herbs and Spices: Showcase how long cooking enables herbs and spices to infuse meals with rich tastes, avoiding the need for excessive salt or harmful additions in recipes.

10. Desserts with a Twist: Surprise readers with slow cooker dessert alternatives, illustrating how this versatile equipment can be utilized to produce healthy sweet delights without losing flavor.

By including slow cooker recipes in the cookbook, readers are offered an extra level of culinary discovery that corresponds with their weight management objectives, making it simpler to maintain a balanced and delicious diet with no effort.

Chapter Four

Seasonal Eating Strategies:

Tailor your meals to the seasons by utilizing locally available food. In spring, appreciate colorful greens like asparagus and peas; summer calls for delicious salads with tomatoes and berries. Fall is great for robust recipes with squash and apples, while winter encourages comforting soups with root vegetables. Seasonal eating increases the freshness, taste, and nutritional value of your meals. Here's a thorough breakdown:

1. Introduction to Seasonal Eating: Begin by discussing the notion of seasonal eating, stressing the benefits of consuming fruits and vegetables when they are naturally in season.

2. Freshness and Flavor: Emphasize how seasonal food tends to be fresher and more tasty, adding to a heightened cooking experience and encouraging readers to enjoy the natural flavors of each component.

3. Nutritional Benefits: Discuss how fruits and vegetables in their prime season frequently claim increased nutritional value. Encourage readers to optimize their intake of vitamins, minerals, and antioxidants by picking fruit that coincides with the current season.

4. Springtime Freshness: Provide dishes that emphasize the brilliant and crisp tastes of spring vegetables, such as asparagus, strawberries, and leafy greens. These meals might include salads, light soups, and foods that embody the spirit of the season.

5. Summer Bounty: Explore dishes that highlight the abundance of summer fruits and vegetables, including tomatoes, berries, corn, and zucchini. Highlight crisp salads, grilled foods, and light dinners suited for warmer weather.

6. Autumn Harvest Feasts: Present substantial meals incorporating the rich tastes of autumn fruit, such as apples, pumpkins, and root vegetables. Include soothing stews, roasted foods, and sweets that reflect the spirit of autumn.

7. Winter Wellness: Showcase dishes that utilize winter veggies like kale, Brussels sprouts, and winter squashes. Emphasize robust and warming meals ideal for winter months, enhancing both taste and nutritional depth.

8. Farmers' Market Inspiration: Encourage readers to visit local farmers' markets and pick products depending on what's in season. Provide suggestions on navigating farmers' markets and planning meals around fresh, locally produced vegetables.

9. Adaptable Seasonal Menus: Offer suggestions on how to adjust current recipes in the cookbook depending on seasonal availability, encouraging flexibility in meal planning and creating a connection with local food cycles.

10. Year-Round Wellness: Conclude by highlighting that seasonal eating is a year-round method to keeping a healthy and diverse diet. Encourage readers to realize the cyclical nature of food supply and its influence on both gastronomic experiences and general well-being.

By embracing seasonal eating practices, the cookbook helps readers not only produce great meals but also develop a connection with the natural cycle of food production, supporting both their taste buds and their health objectives.

Interactive Meal Prepping:

Begin meal planning by picking a range of lean meats, nutritious grains, and colorful veggies. Cook in quantity to generate adaptable components like grilled chicken, quinoa, and roasted vegetables. Divide portions into containers for simple grab-and-go lunches throughout the week. This planned approach to meal preparation encourages weight management by improving portion awareness and limiting the temptation of less nutritious alternatives. Here's a thorough breakdown:

1. Introduction to Meal Preparing: - Begin by describing the idea of meal preparation, highlighting its advantages for weight control, time management, and general convenience.

- Highlight how planning and preparing meals in advance may aid in choosing healthy eating choices and avoiding impulsive selections.

2. Step-by-step advice: - Provide extensive step-by-step advice on how to properly meal prep. Break down the process into simple phases, from organizing the menu to storing cooked meals.

- Include recommendations on choosing a range of nutrient-dense meals, portion management, and balancing macronutrients to support weight control objectives.

3. Menu Planning: - Guide readers in constructing a well-balanced and diversified weekly menu. Encourage the incorporation of a range of fruits, vegetables, lean meats, complete grains, and healthy fats.

- Emphasize the value of integrating bright and tasty components to increase the overall attractiveness of cooked meals.

4. Batch Cooking Techniques: - Explain the notion of batch cooking, where readers may prepare greater amounts of particular components (e.g., grains, proteins) to be utilized in multiple meals throughout the week.

   - Provide recipes that lend themselves nicely to batch cooking and can be readily adapted for several dinners.

5. Interactive Tools and Resources: - Integrate meal-prepping into the meal-prepping instructions, such as downloadable planning templates, checklists, or interactive applications that let readers modify their meal plans based on tastes and dietary restrictions.

6. Storage and Portioning Tips: - Offer practical guidance on correct storage procedures to retain the freshness and quality of preparing meals.

- Guide portioning to ensure that meals correspond with weight management targets, stressing the need for balanced serving sizes.

7. diversity and Flexibility: - Encourage diversity in meal planning to keep things interesting and minimize boredom.
- Highlight the flexibility of meal preparation, enabling readers to alter plans based on changing schedules, tastes, or dietary requirements.

8. Time-Efficient tactics: - Provide time-saving tactics for meal preparation, such as multitasking, utilizing kitchen equipment effectively, and picking dishes that need little cooking time.

- Emphasize that successful meal preparation doesn't have to be time-consuming and can be incorporated into hectic lives.

9. Nutritional advice: - Offer nutritional advice within the meal-preparing guidelines, educate users on choosing nutrient-dense items, and construct meals that support their weight management objectives.

- Address typical nutritional issues and give recommendations on regulating calorie consumption while preserving pleasure and taste.

10. Community Engagement: - Foster a feeling of community by inviting readers to contribute their meal-prepping experiences, recipes, and ideas.

- Provide a platform, whether it's via social media groups or an online community affiliated with the cookbook, where readers can engage, share ideas, and encourage one another in their meal-prepping adventures.

By merging these components into the notion of Interactive Meal Prepping, the cookbook intends to empower readers with practical tools, resources, and advice to make meal planning and preparation an enjoyable and successful part of their weight management approach.

Chapter Six

Flavorful Low-Calorie Desserts:

Indulge your desires with low-calorie treats like fruit skewers drizzled with honey or dark chocolate. Create guilt-free frozen yogurt popsicles with fresh berries. Opt for baked apples with cinnamon or a Greek yogurt parfait with granola and berries. These innovative dishes give pleasant sweetness while fitting with health-conscious ideals. Here's a thorough breakdown:

1. Redefining Dessert Options: - Emphasize the move from conventional, calorie-dense sweets to a new strategy that favors inventive, low-calorie dishes.

- Explain that the objective is to reframe the perspective of desserts, displaying that they can be tasty and rewarding while matching with health and wellness goals.

2. Creative Low-Calorie Recipes:

- Introduce a selection of unique recipes that reinterpret traditional sweets with an emphasis on decreasing total calorie intake.

- Explore novel ingredients and approaches that improve tastes without depending on excessive sugar, fats, or empty calories.

3. Balancing Sweet desires: - Acknowledge the common need for sweet delights and frame low-calorie desserts as a balanced option to fulfill such desires.

- Highlight the use of natural sweeteners, such as stevia, monk fruit, or agave, to deliver sweetness without the extra calories of refined sugars.

4. Health Goals Integration: - Reinforce the concept that these desserts are made to coincide with health goals, such as weight management, by using nutrient-dense foods and attentive portion control.

- Stress the value of eating sweets as part of a well-rounded and balanced diet.

5. deliberate enjoyment: - Encourage a deliberate attitude to enjoyment by enjoying each mouthful of these low-calorie delicacies. Emphasize that it's possible to enjoy dessert without the guilt frequently associated with higher-calorie selections.

6. entire Ingredients Emphasis: - Showcase the use of entire, minimally processed ingredients in crafting low-calorie sweets. This could contain whole grains, nuts, seeds, and fruits that add not just to taste but also to nutritional value.

7. Innovative Flavor Combinations: - Introduce innovative and surprising flavor combinations to enrich the experience of low-calorie sweets. This might entail matching fruits with herbs, experimenting with spices, or introducing unusual ingredients for a blast of flavor.

8. Texture Variation: - Highlight the significance of texture in dessert pleasure. Explore methods to generate pleasing textures without depending on excessive fats or carbohydrates, such as introducing crunchy ingredients like nuts or seeds.

9. Dessert Repurposing: - Provide suggestions for repurposing components often found in desserts into healthier alternatives. For example, converting Greek yogurt into a creamy basis for a fruit parfait or utilizing sweet potatoes in a desert setting.

10. Inclusion of Nutrient-Dense choices: - Integrate nutrient-dense choices into low-calorie desserts to increase their health profile. Consider meals using antioxidant-rich berries, fiber-packed oats, or protein-rich Greek yogurt.

11. Celebration of Seasonal Ingredients: - Encourage the use of seasonal ingredients to improve the freshness and taste of low-calorie sweets. Showcase dishes that coincide with the availability of fruits and tastes throughout the year.

12. User-Friendly Recipes: - Ensure that the recipes are user-friendly, offering clear directions, few materials, and accessible methods to make low-calorie dessert making attainable for a broad variety of home chefs.

By embracing these components, the cookbook intends to reimagine the dessert experience, illustrating that low-calorie choices can be tasty, and gratifying, and contribute to overall health objectives without sacrificing the delight of indulging in sweet sweets.

Chapter Seven

Power of Proteins:

Highlight the value of protein by integrating a range of sources. Include lean meats, poultry, fish, lentils, and plant-based choices like tofu or quinoa in your meals. Recipes such as grilled chicken salads, lentil soups, or chickpea stir-fries highlight varied protein-rich possibilities. Ensuring a sufficient protein intake maintains muscular function, assists in weight control, and adds to a balanced diet overall. Here's a thorough breakdown:

1. Emphasizing Protein Importance: - Start by highlighting the vital function of protein in a balanced diet. Explain that proteins are necessary macronutrients that play a key role in creating and repairing tissues, maintaining immunological function, and providing a source of energy.

2. Protein as a Building Block: - Illustrate how proteins work as building blocks for muscles, bones, skin, and numerous enzymes and hormones in the body.

- Emphasize their relevance in supporting the growth and maintenance of tissues, particularly for persons involved in physical activities or seeking muscular development.

3. Diverse Protein Sources: - Introduce the notion of diversifying protein sources to guarantee a full nutritional intake. Highlight that various protein-rich diets supply differing required amino acids and extra nutrients.

- Promote a combination of animal and plant-based proteins to accommodate varied dietary tastes and demands.

4. Lean Protein Choices: - Encourage the incorporation of lean protein sources in the diet.

Explain the advantages of choosing lean cuts of meat, chicken without skin, fish, tofu, lentils, and low-fat dairy products to decrease saturated fat consumption.

5. Plant-Based Proteins: - Spotlight the relevance of plant-based protein sources for people adopting vegetarian or vegan diets. Showcase protein-rich alternatives including beans, lentils, chickpeas, quinoa, almonds, and seeds.
   - Provide inventive recipes that showcase the protein content of plant-based components.

6. Protein and Weight control: - Discuss the significance of protein in weight control. Explain how proteins contribute to feelings of fullness and aid in controlling appetite, possibly supporting people in obtaining and maintaining a healthy weight.

7. Post-Exercise Recovery: - Highlight the role of protein in post-exercise recovery. Explain that taking protein after physical exercise stimulates muscle repair and development, assisting in overall fitness objectives.

- Provide recipes or meal ideas ideal for post-workout nourishment.

8. Protein-Packed Snack Options:

- Suggest protein-rich snacks to support sustained energy levels throughout the day. This may contain Greek yogurt with fruit, hummus with veggie sticks, or a small handful of almonds.

- Encourage readers to regard snacks as opportunities to integrate more protein into their diet.

9. Unique protein dishes: - Introduce a range of unique dishes that highlight varied protein sources.

This might incorporate inventive preparations of chicken, fish, plant-based burgers, or protein-packed salads.

- Include alternatives that appeal to varied culinary tastes and cultural influences.

10. Protein Beyond Meat: - Expand the awareness of protein sources beyond typical mcat alternatives. Explore fish, eggs, dairy, and plant-based alternatives, giving a wide range of options for various diets.

- Include dishes that showcase the flexibility of different protein sources.

11. Protein in Everyday Meals: - Emphasize the integration of protein into everyday meals, not simply in special or high-protein dishes. Showcase how simple tweaks, such as adding beans to a spaghetti meal or putting grilled chicken into a salad, may improve protein consumption.

12. instructional Components: - Include instructional features inside the cookbook, such as charts or infographics explaining the protein composition of different meals. This helps readers make educated judgments regarding their food choices.

By stressing the Power of Proteins, the cookbook intends to educate readers on the vital function of proteins in their diet, giving practical and enticing recipes that promote a diversified and balanced approach to achieving their protein requirements.

Chapter Eight

Hydration Hacks:

Stay hydrated to promote weight control; try infused water with pieces of citrus fruits, cucumber, and mint for a delicious twist. Herbal teas and coconut water are tasty, low-calorie options. Hydration helps reduce hunger and increases metabolism. Experiment with hydrating dishes to make reaching your regular water consumption pleasurable and beneficial for your weight goals. Here's a thorough breakdown:

1. Understanding the Link Between Hydration and Weight Control: - Start by stressing the relationship between proper hydration and weight control. Explain that being hydrated may help to a healthy metabolism, minimize feelings of hunger, and enhance general well-being.

2. Hydration and Appetite Control: - Discuss how being hydrated might help reduce appetite. Explain that occasionally sensations of thirst may be confused for hunger, and by keeping sufficient water, people may be less likely to consume additional calories via excessive snacking.

3. Role of Water in Metabolism: - Explain the function of water in metabolic processes. Emphasize that appropriate hydration promotes the body's capacity to effectively break down nutrients and transform them into energy, possibly benefiting weight control.

4. Benefits of Hydration for Exercise: - Highlight the necessity of water for people involved in physical activity. Explain that optimal fluid intake enhances endurance, performance, and recovery during exercise, contributing to overall fitness and weight control objectives.

5. Infused Water Recipes: - Introduce a range of infused water recipes to make hydration more fun. Include mixes of fruits, vegetables, and herbs to give a natural taste to water without depending on sugary chemicals.

- Provide suggestions for refreshing combos, such as cucumber-mint, citrus-berry, or watermelon-basil.

6. Hydrating Beverage Options: - Showcase a selection of hydrating drinks beyond ordinary water. Include choices such as herbal teas, coconut water, or sparkling water with a touch of citrus.

- Highlight that hydrating drinks don't have to be restricted to water and may be included in a broad and fun daily routine.

7. Balancing Electrolytes Naturally: - Discuss the need for electrolytes for hydration. Introduce natural sources of electrolytes, such as coconut water, or add a pinch of sea salt to water, to promote hydration and maintain adequate fluid balance.

8. Hydration monitoring Techniques: - Provide techniques for monitoring hydration throughout the day. Encourage readers to utilize tools like water bottles with volume markings, hydration apps, or journaling to track and improve their daily water consumption.

9. adding Hydration into Meals: - Suggest adding hydrating items into meals. Mention that fruits and vegetables with high water content, such as watermelon, cucumber, or lettuce, help with overall hydration and may be excellent complements to meals.

10. Hydration Rituals: - Promote the formation of hydration rituals throughout the day. Encourage readers to form routines like beginning the morning with a glass of water, having a water bottle at their desk, or sipping a hydrating herbal tea in the evening.

11. Customizing Hydration for Preferences: - Recognize that hydration preferences might differ across people. Provide alternatives for still or sparkling water, warm or cold drinks, and a range of flavor profiles to meet various preferences.

12. instructional Components: - Include instructional information on the indicators of dehydration, the relevance of urine color as an indicator of hydration status, and advice for daily water consumption depending on individual requirements.

By studying Hydration Hacks, the cookbook intends to educate readers on the relevance of being hydrated for weight control and general health. Through infused water recipes, hydrating beverage alternatives, and practical recommendations, it promotes the implementation of good hydration practices into everyday life.

Chapter Nine

Smart Substitutions:

Optimize recipes by switching items to cut calories and fat. Replace oil with applesauce in baking, use Greek yogurt instead of sour cream, and pick healthful grains over processed ones. Incorporating clever replacements, such as utilizing herbs for flavor or lighter meats, preserves taste while keeping with calorie-conscious aims. Small modifications may have a major influence on the nutritional composition of your favorite recipes. Here's a thorough breakdown:

1. Introduction to Smart replacements: - Begin by highlighting the concept that adopting clever ingredient replacements may drastically lower calorie and fat content in dishes while retaining the exquisite flavor.

- Highlight that these alternatives provide a healthier option without reducing the overall pleasure of the meal.

2. Calorie and Fat Reduction Goals:
   - Communicate the major aims of smart substitutions: decreasing total calorie and fat consumption without compromising taste or enjoyment.
   - Emphasize that simple modifications in components may lead to healthy eating habits and assist weight control objectives.

3. Ingredient Swaps for Calorie Reduction:
   - Provide a list of typical ingredient replacements that may lower calorie content. For example, using Greek yogurt instead of sour cream, applesauce instead of oil, or whole wheat flour instead of refined flour.
   - Explain the calorie differences between the original and replacement components.

4. Healthy Fat Alternatives: - Introduce alternatives to saturated fats that keep flavor while supporting heart health. Examples include substituting butter with avocado, using olive oil instead of solid fats, or integrating nuts and seeds for extra texture and healthy fats.

5. Balancing Nutritional Value: - Emphasize the necessity of preserving or boosting the nutritional value of a meal via judicious alternatives. For instance, substituting white rice with cauliflower rice to enhance vegetable consumption or integrating quinoa for extra protein.

6. Sweeteners and Sugar Alternatives: - Discuss alternatives to refined sugars for people wishing to limit their sugar consumption. This might involve utilizing natural sweeteners like honey, maple syrup, or stevia, or adding fruits for sweetness.
   - Guide on altering sweetness levels depending on personal tastes.

7. Texture and taste Preservation: - Highlight the importance of texture and taste while making substitutes. Ensure that the suggested alternatives preserve or improve the intended texture and taste characteristics of the original recipe.

- Provide ideas on striking the proper balance to avoid compromising the whole eating experience.

8. Allergen-Friendly replacements: - Address common allergies by offering allergen-friendly replacements. For example, providing dairy-free alternatives for people with lactose intolerance or proposing gluten-free choices for persons with gluten sensitivity.

- Ensure that the substitutes retain the integrity of the meal.

9. Recipe-Specific Substitution Tips:

- Offer substitute recommendations customized to certain sorts of dishes.

For instance, advise on healthier alternatives for baking, cooking, or producing dressings and sauces.

- Provide insights on which substitutes work well for particular culinary applications.

10. instructional Components: - Include instructional pieces highlighting the nutritional advantages of wise substitutes. Help readers comprehend the influence of ingredient selections on their overall health and well-being.

- Provide other information or references for further investigation of healthy ingredient replacements.

11. Cooking and Baking skills: - Offer insights into cooking and baking skills that support wise alternatives. For instance, recommendations on altering oven temperatures, mixing procedures, or cooking periods to suit variations in components.

12. Community Engagement: - Foster a feeling of community by inviting readers to share their experiences with smart substitutes. Create a venue for discussing ideas, techniques, and success stories relating to healthy cooking and eating habits.

By offering Smart Substitutions, the cookbook strives to equip readers with practical information and tools for choosing sensible ingredient choices. It gives a path for decreasing calorie and fat content without affecting the flavor and pleasure of their favorite recipes.

Chapter Ten

Weekend Indulgences:

Savor guilt-free weekend indulgences with dishes like dark chocolate-dipped strawberries or homemade granola bars. Opt for complete components and careful quantities to enjoy without derailing your balanced approach to weight management. These occasional snacks may be both rewarding and delightful without sacrificing your overall health objectives. Here's a thorough breakdown:

1. Introduction to Weekend Indulgences: - Start by outlining the rationale behind Weekend Indulgences. Emphasize that these recipes are meant to enable guilt-free enjoyment of goodies, knowing that occasional indulgences may be part of a balanced approach to weight management.

2. Occasional Indulgences in a Balanced Diet: - Reinforce the concept that occasional indulgences may be included in a balanced and healthy eating routine. Emphasize the value of balance and conscious pleasure to prevent emotions of guilt or restriction.

3. Weekend as a Special Occasion: - Position the weekend as a special occasion for savoring pleasures. Encourage readers to regard weekend indulgences as a reward for maintaining a health-conscious attitude during the week rather than a deviation from their objectives.

4. Guilt-Free Approach: - Highlight the notion of guilt-free pleasures. Explain that the dishes included in this area are created to eliminate needless calories, carbohydrates, and fats while enhancing taste and enjoyment.

   - Reinforce the concept that consuming goodies should be a positive and joyful experience.

5. Balancing Portion amounts: - Guide balancing portion amounts for weekend indulgences. Encourage readers to relish smaller quantities of delicious meals, allowing them pleasure without excessive calorie consumption.

6. unique and delectable foods: - Showcase a range of unique and delectable foods that are normally associated with weekends. This might include baked goods, pastries, or nibbles that convey a feeling of celebration and relaxation.
   - Feature recipes that employ clever replacements to lower calorie and fat levels while keeping the enjoyment of the treat.

7. Nutrient-Dense components: - Introduce nutrient-dense components in indulgent meals to increase their overall health profile. For example, integrating entire grains, fruits, or nuts to provide nutritional benefits while keeping flavor.

8. participatory Preparation: - Encourage a participatory and engaging approach to preparing weekend pleasures. Include advice on integrating family or friends in the culinary process, turning it into a shared and joyful experience.

9. Seasonal and Festive Treats: - Align weekend excesses with seasonal or festive themes. Provide recipes that represent the tastes and ingredients associated with holidays or special events, heightening the feeling of excitement and celebration.

10. Mindful Eating habits: - Introduce mindful eating habits for weekend goodies. Encourage readers to relish each mouthful, paying attention to tastes, textures, and overall delight. This might improve the enjoyment gained from indulgences.

11. Physical Activity Integration: - Suggest incorporating physical activity into weekend habits. Emphasize that being active may help to a balanced approach to weight management and give a good outlet for enjoying pleasures.

12. Community Sharing and Feedback: - Foster a feeling of community by inviting readers to share their experiences with Weekend Indulgences. Create a forum for sharing photographs, advice, and variants, enabling readers to encourage and support one another.

By presenting Weekend Indulgences in this manner, the cookbook intends to alter the view of occasional sweets, making them a positive and joyful component of balanced living. The recipes presented provide a guilt-free approach to weekend pleasures, enabling readers to relish the moment while keeping their overall health objectives.

Chapter Eleven

Portion Control Tips:

Master portion management by using smaller dishes, measuring serving sizes, and splitting snacks into separate amounts. Visuhealthyalize correct portions - a serving of protein is around the size of your hand. Fill half your plate with vegetables and split the remaining space for carbohydrates and meats. These practical suggestions and visual signals enable you to maintain a balance in your meals. Here's a thorough breakdown:

1. Importance of Portion Control: - Start by highlighting the necessity of portion management in maintaining a healthy balance. Explain that it plays a critical role in controlling calorie intake, supporting weight management, and boosting general well-being.

2. Caloric Awareness: - Educate readers about the link between portion sizes and calorie consumption. Help them realize that being more conscious of portion sizes is a critical step toward making educated and mindful eating choices.

3. Visual Guides and Comparisons: - Provide visual tips and comparisons to assist readers in better grasping acceptable portion amounts. Use ordinary items or visual cues, such as a deck of cards for a dish of meat or a tennis ball for a meal of pasta, to make portion management more apparent.

4. Handy measuring procedures: - Introduce practical measuring procedures that don't need kitchen utensils. For example, using the hand as a reference for serving sizes: the palm for protein, the fist for vegetables, the cupped hand for carbs, and the thumb for fats.

5. Plate Composition ways: - Offer ways for building well-balanced plates. Encourage readers to envision splitting their plate into quarters, designating a portion for protein, veggies, whole grains, and healthy fats to make a balanced and nutritious meal.

6. Mindful Eating habits: - Promote mindful eating habits as a supplement to portion control. Encourage readers to eat slowly, appreciate each mouthful, and pay attention to hunger and fullness indicators, allowing for a more mindful and pleasurable eating experience.

7. Pre-Portioned Snacks: - Suggest pre-portioned snacks as an easy approach to reduce calorie consumption. Provide suggestions for assembling snack packs with nuts, fruits, or cut-up veggies, making it easy for readers to take a tasty and regulated quantity.

8. Plate Size and Serveware Selection: - Discuss the influence of plate size and serveware on perceived portion sizes. Highlight that using smaller plates and bowls may generate an optical illusion, making servings look bigger and thus leading to greater pleasure with fewer quantities of food.

9. Meal Planning for Portion Control: - Guide readers in adopting portion control into their meal planning. Provide ideas on preparing meals in advance, utilizing containers to divide out portions, and having a clear strategy for balanced and regulated eating throughout the day.

10. Listen to Hunger and Fullness Signals: - Encourage readers to listen to their hunger and fullness cues. Emphasize the significance of quitting eating when full rather than completing what's on the plate, even if there's still food left.

11. Nutrient-Dense Choices: - Highlight the notion of selecting nutrient-dense meals to increase nutritional benefit within restricted quantities. Encourage readers to concentrate on foods rich in vitamins, minerals, and other critical nutrients for optimum wellness.

12. Community Support and Accountability: - Foster a feeling of community support by inviting readers to share their portion control tactics and triumphs. Create a place for debates, exchanging suggestions, and celebrating successes related to mastering portion management.

By giving practical Portion Control Tips and visual guidelines, the cookbook strives to enable readers to make educated decisions about their food quantities. The objective is to help them create persistent habits that lead to a healthy and balanced approach to eating.

Chapter Twelve

Balanced Breakfast Bonanza:

Kickstart your day with a nutritious breakfast; try oatmeal with fruits and nuts, a veggie-packed omelet, or Greek yogurt with granola. These dishes include a balance of complex carbohydrates, protein, and healthy fats to power your morning and support your weight goals. Experiment with varied alternatives to keep your breakfasts both healthful and delicious. Here's a thorough breakdown:

1. Importance of a Nutritious Breakfast: - Begin by highlighting the value of beginning the day with a healthy meal. Explain that a balanced morning meal delivers critical nutrients, raises energy levels, and sets a favorable tone for the remainder of the day.

2. Fueling and Supporting Weight Goals: - Highlight the function of a nutritious meal in feeding the body and supporting weight-related objectives. Emphasize that a well-constructed morning meal may lead to fullness, minimizing the chance of overeating later in the day.

3. Variety in Breakfast Options: - Showcase a broad choice of breakfast dishes to accommodate various tastes and dietary concerns. Include alternatives that contain whole grains, lean meats, healthy fats, and a range of fruits and vegetables.

4. Nutrient-Dense items: - Introduce nutrient-dense items to increase the nutritional profile of breakfast meals. This can include whole grains like oats or quinoa, protein sources such as eggs or Greek yogurt, and fiber-rich fruits and vegetables.

5. Balancing Macronutrients: - Guide readers on balancing macronutrients in their breakfast. Encourage a balance of carbs, proteins, and fats to offer continuous energy, improve muscular function, and add to overall enjoyment.

6. Quick and simple alternatives: - Include quick and simple breakfast alternatives for hectic mornings. Provide dishes that may be made ahead of time or assembled quickly, so that time restrictions don't impede the ability to start the day with a nutritious meal.

7. Customizable Breakfast Bowls: - Inspire the construction of personalized breakfast bowls. Offer several foundation alternatives including yogurt, oats, or smoothie bases, and present a selection of toppings such as nuts, seeds, fruits, and granola to enable readers to build their breakfast to their tastes.

8. Protein-Packed Morning Options: - Showcase protein-packed breakfast alternatives to encourage satiety and muscular support. This might incorporate meals using eggs, dairy, plant-based proteins, or adding protein-rich grains like quinoa into morning dishes.

9. Whole Food Sweeteners: - Introduce whole food sweeteners as alternatives in breakfast meals. Encourage the use of naturally sweet products such as honey, maple syrup, or mashed bananas to enhance sweetness without depending on refined sugars.

10. Incorporating Superfoods: - Explore the inclusion of superfoods into breakfast dishes for extra nutritional advantages. This may contain nutrients like chia seeds, flaxseeds, berries, or green leafy vegetables that deliver an additional burst of vitamins, minerals, and antioxidants.

11. Balanced Breakfast Smoothies: - Provide suggestions for balanced breakfast smoothies. Emphasize the mix of fruits, vegetables, proteins, and healthy fats to make smoothies that are not only tasty but also nutrient-dense.

12. Community Sharing and Feedback: - Foster a feeling of community by asking readers to share their favorite balanced breakfast recipes. Create a forum for sharing photographs, recipes, and suggestions, enabling readers to encourage and support one another in their breakfast choices.

By offering a Balanced Breakfast Bonanza, the cookbook intends to motivate readers to make educated and health-conscious decisions at the beginning of their day. The recipes presented are meant to be not just healthy and tasty but also varied and adaptable to individual tastes and dietary objectives.

Chapter Thirteen

Global Fusion Fitness Menu:

Infuse global tastes into fitness-oriented meals by blending spices and ingredients from diverse cuisines. Try a Thai-inspired quinoa salad with peanut sauce or a Mediterranean-style grilled chicken with tzatziki. These fusion recipes not only bring excitement to your fitness menu but also give a varied variety of nutrients to help your health and wellness quest. Here's a thorough breakdown:

1. Culinary variety: - Emphasize the culinary variety contained in the Global Fusion Fitness Menu. The objective is to blend tastes, ingredients, and culinary methods from many cuisines globally, producing a rich and intriguing tapestry of taste.

2. Integration of Global tastes: - Showcase the integration of global tastes into fitness-oriented meals. This entails combining ingredients from Mediterranean, Asian, Latin American, Middle Eastern, and other cuisines to provide depth and diversity to the meal.

3. Balanced Nutrition: - Reinforce the commitment to balanced nutrition within fitness-oriented meals. The combination of world tastes should not only increase taste but also add to a well-rounded and nutrient-dense eating experience, supporting fitness objectives.

4. Incorporating Lean Proteins: - Highlight the integration of lean protein sources from varied ethnic cuisines. This could mean combining fish, chicken, lentils, tofu, or other protein-rich items served with global-inspired tastes and cooking techniques.

5. Whole Grains and Complex Carbs: - Showcase the usage of whole grains and complex carbs in fitness-oriented meals. Introduce grains like quinoa, brown rice, or farro, borrowing inspiration from world cuisines that have long exploited these nutrient-rich mainstays.

6. Abundant Vegetables and Plant-Based Components: - Emphasize the availability of vegetables and plant-based components in the Global Fusion Fitness Menu. Explore colorful and savory alternatives inspired by various cuisines to encourage a diversified and plant-centric approach to fitness eating.

7. Smart Fats and Healthy Oils: - Incorporate smart fats and healthy oils into the cuisine. Showcase the use of olive oil, avocado, nuts, and seeds—drawing influence from the Mediterranean and other cuisines recognized for their focus on heart-healthy fats.

8. Culinary skills from throughout the globe:
- Introduce culinary skills and practices from throughout the globe. This could involve stir-frying, grilling, roasting, or slow-cooking, tailored to fitness-oriented meals to improve tastes without sacrificing nutritional objectives.

9. Balancing Spices and Herbs: - Explore the technique of balancing spices and herbs to boost the flavor of fitness meals. Draw inspiration from numerous regional spice mixes and herb combinations that not only provide taste but also contribute to the antioxidant and anti-inflammatory characteristics of the food.

10. Global-Inspired Fitness Bowls: - Feature fitness bowls that bring together ingredients from various corners of the globe. These might include grain bowls, poke bowls, or Buddha bowls, each expressing a fusion of flavors and textures influenced by world culinary traditions.

11. Hybrid Snack and Meal choices: - Introduce hybrid snack and meal choices that smoothly integrate worldwide cuisines. This might entail crafting fitness-friendly versions of foreign street food or snacks that take influence from other cuisines.

12. Cultural background and Education: - Provide cultural background and educational insights into the origin of products, recipes, and culinary processes. This not only improves the gastronomic experience but also creates a respect for the worldwide variety reflected in the fitness-oriented cuisine.

By designing the Global Fusion Fitness Menu, the cookbook intends to deliver a gastronomic adventure that goes beyond standard fitness meals. It attempts to encourage folks to experience a diverse assortment of tastes, textures, and ingredients from across the globe while aligning with their fitness and health objectives. The marriage of flavor and health in this menu strives to make fitness-oriented dining a pleasurable and internationally inspired-experience.

Chapter Fourteen

One-Pan Wonders:

Streamline dinner with one-pan marvels; throw vegetables, lean meats, and spices on a baking sheet for a hassle-free but delectable feast. Opt for meals like roasted chicken with veggies or sheet pan fajitas to ease both preparation and cleaning. These practical solutions coincide with a weight-conscious lifestyle without sacrificing flavor. Here's a thorough breakdown:

1. Streamlining Meal Preparation: - Highlight the fundamental purpose of One-Pan Wonders: streamlining meal preparation. Explain that these recipes are meant to decrease the amount of dishes and tasks required, making cooking more efficient and accessible.

2. Efficient cleaning: - Emphasize the efficiency of cleaning related to one-pan recipes. By utilizing a single pan for the whole meal, users may considerably minimize the time and effort spent on cleaning dishes, matching the convenience demands of a busy lifestyle.

3. Weight-Conscious Lifestyle Integration: - Integrate the notion of One-Pan Wonders into a weight-conscious lifestyle. Emphasize that these recipes are created to correspond with health and weight management objectives, containing balanced and healthy components while simplifying the whole cooking procedure.

4. Balanced Nutrient Profiles: - Reinforce the commitment to balanced nutritional profiles within one-pan meals. Ensure that the meals feature a combination of lean meats, nutritious grains, and a range of veggies to create a thorough and fulfilling eating experience.

5. flexibility of Ingredients: - Showcase the flexibility of ingredients within one-pan dishes. Explain that people may personalize these meals depending on their tastes and dietary needs, providing flexibility while maintaining a weight-conscious approach.

6. innovative Seasoning and Flavor Profiles: - Introduce innovative seasoning and flavor profiles to improve the taste of one-pan dishes. Explore the use of herbs, spices, and marinades to provide depth and diversity without the need for additional pots and pans.

7. Time-saving procedures: - Provide time-saving procedures linked with one-pan cooking. This could involve methods like preparing items in advance, utilizing pre-cut veggies, or selecting quick-cooking meats to expedite the whole cooking procedure.

8. Meal-Prepping options: - Highlight the meal-prepping options that one-pan dishes provide. These recipes may be favorable to batch cooking, enabling users to make bigger amounts and have ready-made meals for the week, supporting a regular and weight-conscious eating plan.

9. Incorporating entire products: - Emphasize the use of entire, minimally processed products in one-pan dishes. This not only adds to the nutritional worth of the meals but also corresponds with a weight-conscious lifestyle that stresses healthful food choices.

10. Balancing Macronutrients: - Guide folks on balancing macronutrients within one-pan meals. Emphasize the necessity of adding protein, healthy fats, and carbs in proper quantities to make tasty and well-rounded foods.

11. Interactive Cooking Experience: - Encourage an interactive cooking experience with one-pan recipes. Whether for solitary chefs or families, underline that the simplicity of these recipes provides for a more joyful and stress-free time in the kitchen.

12. Community Sharing and Variation: - Foster a feeling of community by asking readers to contribute their favorite versions and adaptations of one-pan recipes. Create a venue for discussing advice, success stories, and creative tweaks on these basic but delectable foods.

By providing One-Pan Wonders, the cookbook strives to make healthy and weight-conscious eating more accessible and practical. The emphasis on simplicity, efficiency, and balanced nutrition corresponds with the demands of those seeking simple and tasty meal alternatives without sacrificing their health and fitness objectives.

Chapter Fifteen

Herbs and Spices for Health:

Harness the therapeutic capabilities of herbs and spices by including turmeric in curries for its anti-inflammatory effects or adding cinnamon to porridge to help manage blood sugar. Experiment with using rosemary in roasted meals for antioxidant benefits. By infusing your meals with these delectable additives, you not only boost taste but also contribute to general well-being. Here's a thorough breakdown:

1. Introduction to Medicinal Properties: - Start by conveying the concept that herbs and spices go beyond tasting; they contain healing characteristics. Explain that numerous herbs and spices have been historically utilized for their possible health advantages, ranging from anti-inflammatory to antioxidant characteristics.

2. Diverse Culinary and Medicinal Uses: - Showcase the variety of herbs and spices in both culinary and medicinal settings. Provide examples of herbs like basil, rosemary, and thyme, as well as spices such as turmeric, cinnamon, and ginger, each having distinct taste profiles and possible health-promoting properties.

3. Adding functional components: - Emphasize the notion of adding functional components into everyday meals. Showcase how combining herbs and spices into dishes, not only boosts taste but also helps general well-being, encouraging a holistic approach to health.

4. Antioxidant-Rich Options: - Highlight herbs and spices recognized for their antioxidant-rich characteristics. For example, study how oregano, cinnamon, and cloves might assist in neutralizing free radicals in the body, possibly aiding in cellular health and lowering oxidative stress.

5. Anti-Inflammatory Choices: - Explore anti-inflammatory herbs and spices that may be effortlessly included in meals. Discuss how substances like turmeric, ginger, and garlic have been historically utilized for their possible anti-inflammatory benefits, promoting joint and general health.

6. Digestive Health Enhancement: - Introduce herbs and spices recognized for their favorable effects on digestion. Discuss the addition of peppermint, fennel, and coriander, which may assist in digestive comfort and contribute to a healthy gut.

7. Adapting Traditional Healing Practices: - Explore how the use of herbs and spices for health is rooted in ancient medicinal techniques. Discuss how civilizations across the globe have traditionally exploited these natural substances not just for culinary reasons but also as cures for different health concerns.

8. Heart-Healthy Choices: - Spotlight herbs and spices connected with heart health. For instance, highlight how garlic, cayenne pepper, and cinnamon may have cardiovascular advantages, such as promoting healthy blood pressure and cholesterol levels.

9. Mindful Flavoring for Reduced Sodium: - Encourage the conscious use of herbs and spices as alternatives to excessive salt. Discuss how including tasty alternatives like basil, thyme, and rosemary may boost taste without depending on high amounts of salt, contributing to heart-healthy eating.

10. Balancing Sweet and Savory with Spices:
- Explore the balance between sweet and savory tastes with spices. Discuss how cinnamon, nutmeg, and cardamom may provide warmth and sweetness to recipes without depending on excessive sugar, contributing to a more health-conscious approach to sweetness.

11. Interactive Cooking Demonstrations: - Offer interactive cooking demonstrations that illustrate the inclusion of herbs and spices for both taste and health advantages. Provide practical ideas on how to enhance the therapeutic benefits of these products throughout the cooking process.

12. Educational Resources and References: - Include educational components inside the cookbook, such as a lexicon of herbs and spices, their health advantages, and references to scientific research supporting their possible therapeutic capabilities.

This provides readers with the knowledge to make educated decisions about the substances they use.

By addressing the notion of Herbs and Spices for Health, the cookbook attempts to motivate readers to regard these substances not just as taste enhancers but also as vital contributors to their general well-being. The incorporation of herbs and spices into dishes creates a comprehensive approach to culinary delight and health enhancement.

Chapter Sixteen

Social Dining Strategies:

Navigate social situations by selecting smaller amounts, choosing grilled or steamed alternatives, and being cautious of liquid calories. Share meals to limit quantities and emphasize vegetables. When eating out, aim for lean protein and veggie-based selections. Prepare for gatherings by having a nutritious snack beforehand to prevent overindulging. These tactics let you enjoy social meals while keeping connected with your weight control objectives. Here's a thorough breakdown:

1. Navigating Social events: - Start by addressing the issues people may have while attending social events while aiming to maintain weight control objectives. Acknowledge the availability of enticing food alternatives and the associated pressure to indulge.

2. thoughtful Decision-Making: - Emphasize the significance of thoughtful decision-making in social contexts. Encourage readers to approach social meals with a proactive perspective, making mindful choices that correspond with their health aims while still enjoying the event.

3. ways for Buffets and Events: - Provide realistic ways for handling buffet-style events. Offer ideas on examining all available alternatives before choosing a plate, concentrating on lesser servings, and emphasizing entire, nutrient-dense meals.

4. Pre-Eating Strategies: - Discuss the notion of pre-eating before social gatherings to prevent excessive hunger.

Suggest eating a healthy and fulfilling lunch or snack beforehand to help regulate quantities and limit the temptation to overindulge.

5. Balancing Alcohol Consumption: - Address the influence of alcohol on weight control. Offer tactics for controlling alcohol consumption during social events, such as choosing lighter beverages, interspersing drinks with water, and establishing boundaries to minimize extra calorie intake.

6. Mindful Eating Strategies: - Introduce mindful eating strategies for social dining. Encourage readers to appreciate each mouthful, eat carefully, and pay attention to hunger and fullness indicators, encouraging a more mindful and pleasurable dining experience.

7. Healthy Potluck Contributions: - Provide suggestions for presenting healthy meals to potluck-style parties.
Share recipes that are both tasty and healthy, ensuring there are alternatives accessible that correspond with weight control objectives.

8. Restaurant-Friendly meals: - Include a range of restaurant-friendly meals that consumers may prepare at home before eating out. These recipes may be customized to resemble famous restaurant meals, delivering healthier options while enabling consumers to experience their favorite tastes.

9. browsing Restaurant Menus: - Offer suggestions for browsing restaurant menus while making health-conscious decisions. Encourage readers to search for grilled or baked alternatives, pick lean meats, choose vegetable sides, and be mindful of portion sizes.

10. Communication tactics: - Discuss effective communication tactics for dietary preferences or limits while attending social activities. Empower readers to convey their demands appropriately, whether it's asking for alterations at a restaurant or notifying hosts about dietary restrictions.

11. Community Support and Accountability:
- Foster a feeling of community support by inviting readers to share their social eating tactics and success stories. Create a venue for discussing insights, challenges, and support to handle social settings while sticking to weight control objectives.

12. Celebrating Without Guilt: - Reinforce the concept that social meals are about celebration and pleasure. Guide readers to achieve a balance between relishing special moments, making attentive decisions, and avoiding feelings of guilt connected with occasional excesses.

By presenting Social Dining Strategies, the cookbook attempts to equip readers to navigate social settings without sacrificing their weight control objectives. The combination of practical suggestions, mindful eating practices, and restaurant-friendly dishes gives a holistic strategy for enjoying social occasions while keeping a healthy lifestyle.

Chapter Seventeen

Fiber-Rich Feast:

Craft a fiber-rich feast with dishes like lentil and vegetable stew, quinoa salads with a range of colorful vegetables, and chia seed pudding for dessert. High-fiber meals enhance satiety, help in weight control, and contribute to digestive health. Including a range of fiber sources in your meals guarantees a full and healthful feast. Here's a thorough breakdown:

1. Celebrating the Benefits of Fiber: - Begin by highlighting the significance and advantages of dietary fiber, not only for digestive health but also for its involvement in weight control. Highlight that a fiber-rich diet may lead to a sensation of fullness, assisting in appetite management.

2. Understanding Dietary Fiber: - Provide a summary of dietary fiber, noting that it covers plant-based carbohydrates that the body cannot digest. Mention the two major types: soluble fiber, which dissolves in water, and insoluble fiber, which adds weight to the diet.

3. Satiety and Weight Management: - Explore how fiber improves satiety and weight control. Discuss how high-fiber meals take longer to chew and digest, generating a sensation of fullness that may lead to lower total calorie intake, thus supporting weight management objectives.

4. Digestive Health Promotion: - Emphasize the function of fiber in supporting digestive health. Discuss how fiber adds weight to stool, assists in regular bowel movements, and contributes to a healthy gut microbiota, encouraging a balanced and efficient digestive system.

5. Whole Food Fiber Sources: - Showcase a range of whole food sources high in fiber. Include fruits, vegetables, whole grains, legumes, nuts, and seeds, highlighting the range of alternatives available for people to integrate into their diets.

6. Balanced Fiber Intake: - Guide readers on obtaining a balanced intake of both soluble and insoluble fiber. Emphasize that a diversified and well-rounded diet that incorporates multiple fiber sources may give a larger variety of health advantages.

7. Interactive Meal Planning: - Encourage an interactive approach to meal planning with an emphasis on fiber-rich items. Provide advice on making meals that incorporate a combination of fiber sources, delivering a pleasurable and nutrient-dense dining experience.

8. Fiber-Rich Recipe characteristics: - Introduce unique characteristics of dishes inside the Fiber-Rich Feast area. Emphasize that each dish is intended to be not only tasty but also filled with fiber, highlighting the adaptability of high-fiber products.

9. adding Fiber into Every Meal: - Guide on adding fiber into every meal, from breakfast to supper. Offer suggestions for adding fruits, vegetables, whole grains, and legumes to diverse recipes to enhance total fiber consumption.

10. Meal Prep with Fiber in Mind: - Suggest meal prep tactics that highlight fiber-rich products. Provide insights into batch-cooking fiber-packed components, such as roasted vegetables, whole grains, or legume-based recipes, for simple incorporation into meals throughout the week.

11. Fiber and taste Pairings: - Explore pairings of fiber-rich products that not only give health advantages but also enrich the taste profile of meals. For example, mixing fruits with yogurt, putting nuts and seeds into salads, or adding beans to soups and stews.

12. Community Sharing and Success Stories: - Foster a feeling of community by asking readers to share their experiences with adding more fiber into their diets. Create a forum for sharing success stories, favorite recipes, and strategies for making fiber-rich nutrition pleasurable and sustainable.

By presenting the Fiber-Rich Feast, the cookbook intends to promote the good influence of fiber on both satiety and digestive health. The featured recipes are aimed to encourage readers to enjoy a variety of tasty meals that contribute to their overall well-being and weight control objectives.

Chapter Eighteen

Family Fitness Challenges:

Engage in family fitness challenges with events like weekend walks, dance-offs, or friendly sports tournaments. Accompany them with nutritious meals, such as fruit smoothie bowls or whole-grain wraps, to encourage a healthy and active lifestyle. Combining exciting challenges with nourishing meals develops a feeling of connection while encouraging overall family well-being. Here's a thorough breakdown:

1. Promoting a Healthy, Active Lifestyle: - Start by highlighting the necessity of creating a healthy and active lifestyle among families. Highlight the advantages of regular physical exercise for both adults and children, including better fitness, mood, and general well-being.

2. Family Bonding via Fitness: - Introduce the notion that fitness challenges may be a fun and participatory method for families to connect. Explain that engaging in activities together not only boosts physical health but also enhances the emotional relationships within the family unit.

3. range of Fitness tasks: - Showcase a range of fitness tasks ideal for various fitness levels and ages. This might include outdoor activities, home exercises, friendly contests, and team-based challenges, providing inclusion and involvement for all family members.

4. creating reasonable objectives: - Emphasize the significance of creating reasonable fitness objectives for family challenges.

Discuss how these challenges may be adjusted to individual capacities, giving a feeling of achievement and inspiration to continue the road toward a healthy lifestyle.

5. Creating a pleasant atmosphere: - Discuss the need to establish a pleasant and supportive atmosphere during family fitness challenges. Emphasize that the main purpose is to have fun together, developing a spirit of collaboration and encouragement rather than focusing simply on competition.

6. Interactive Fitness Calendar: - Introduce the notion of an interactive fitness calendar. Provide a roadmap for families to plan and monitor their fitness challenges throughout time, giving a visual depiction of their successes and development.

7. Nutritious Recipes to Complement Fitness: - Connect fitness challenges with nutritional foods that complement an active lifestyle.

Offer a range of dishes intended to offer the energy and nutrition required for physical exercise, stressing the necessity of fuelling the body with nutritious foods.

8. Post-Challenge Recovery Meals: - Provide suggestions for post-challenge recovery meals. Highlight the necessity of replenishing energy reserves and promoting muscle repair with meals that contain a mix of protein, carbs, and healthy fats.

9. Incorporating Family-Friendly Activities: - Include family-friendly activities that integrate exercise with fun. This might be hiking, bicycling, swimming, dance parties, or simply innovative games that get everyone moving and laughing together.

10. Fitness Challenges for Various Ages: - Tailor exercise challenges to suit different age groups within the family.

Provide adaptations for younger children, ensuring that challenges are age-appropriate and pleasant for everyone.

11. Educational Components: - Include educational components inside the fitness tasks. Share information on the advantages of many forms of activities, the necessity of being hydrated, and advice for maintaining a healthy and active lifestyle.

12. Community Sharing and Celebrations: - Foster a feeling of community among families participating in the challenges. Encourage sharing experiences, images, and success stories on a dedicated platform, building a supportive network for celebrating triumphs and conquering problems.

By providing Family Fitness Challenges mixed with healthy dishes, the cookbook intends to motivate families to go on a path toward a better and more active lifestyle together. The focus on fun, inclusion, and positive reinforcement creates an atmosphere where exercise becomes a shared and joyful family activity.

Chapter Nineteen

Mindful Eating Journal:

Initiate a mindful eating diary to note behaviors, feelings, and progress. Note what you eat, when, and how you feel. Reflect on portion amounts and hunger levels. This exercise increases awareness, helping spot trends and make educated decisions on your weight control path. Regularly rereading your notebook may give significant insights and promote good adjustments in your eating habits. Here's a thorough breakdown:

1. Purpose of Mindful Eating Journal: - Start by describing the objective of the mindful eating notebook. Emphasize that it acts as a tool for self-reflection, helping readers build awareness of their eating patterns, emotional triggers, and overall success on their weight control journey.

2. Tracking Eating patterns: - Encourage readers to use the notebook to document their eating patterns. This involves tracking meals, snacks, portion sizes, and the time of their eating. The idea is to build an awareness of what, when, and how much they are eating.

3. Emotional Eating Awareness: - Highlight the importance of the mindful eating diary in developing awareness of emotional eating. Encourage readers to record their emotional state before, during, and after meals, helping them uncover trends and triggers linked to stress, boredom, or other emotions.

4. Sensory Experience documenting: - Suggest documenting the sensory experience of each meal. Encourage readers to pay attention to the flavor, texture, and scent of their meal.

This technique fosters a more thoughtful and joyful eating experience, developing a connection with the sensory qualities of food.

5. Physical Hunger and Fullness: - Guide readers to listen to their bodily hunger and fullness signals. Encourage children to rate their hunger and fullness levels before and after meals on a scale, promoting a stronger awareness of when to eat and when to quit.

6. Mindful Eating strategies: - Provide suggestions or recommendations for implementing mindful eating strategies into the notebook. This might include behaviors like eating without interruptions, enjoying each mouthful, and taking breaks between meals to check in with feelings of satisfaction.

7. Goal Setting and Progress Tracking: - Introduce areas in the notebook for setting realistic objectives linked to mindful eating and weight control. Encourage readers to monitor their progress over time, recognizing triumphs and revising objectives as appropriate.

8. Reflection on Food Choices: - Prompt readers to reflect on their food choices. This might entail examining the nutritional content of meals, reviewing the balance of food categories, and finding areas where better choices can be made without compromising pleasure.

9. Meal Planning and Preparation comments: - Include room for comments on meal planning and preparation. This might help readers organize their approach to meals, plan for balanced nutrition, and reflect on the work they put into making healthful and enjoyable cuisine.

10. thanks and Positive Affirmations: - Encourage the habit of expressing thanks for meals and fostering positive affirmations. Prompt readers to realize the nutrients their bodies get and embrace the path toward healthy eating habits.

11. Behavioral Patterns Analysis: - Guide readers to study behavioral patterns connected to eating. This involves recognizing circumstances or locations where they may confront problems and creating solutions to manage such times wisely.

12. Community Sharing and Support: - Foster a feeling of community by inviting readers to contribute ideas, problems, and accomplishments from their mindful eating journey. Provide a venue for them to network, share advice, and provide support to one another.

By adding a thoughtful Eating Journal, the cookbook intends to enable readers to adopt a thoughtful and purposeful attitude to eating. The diary serves as a helpful tool for self-discovery, helping people make mindful decisions that match their weight management and general well-being objectives.

Chapter Twenty

Kitchen Confidence Workshops:

Empower kitchen confidence with virtual or in-person seminars. Cover fundamental culinary skills, ingredient substitutions, and recipe modification. Encourage individuals to ask questions and share their experiences. By enhancing culinary abilities, you enable people to take charge of their eating, encouraging a beneficial influence on their weight management journey. Here's a thorough breakdown:

1. purpose of the Workshops: - Start by describing the major purpose of the Kitchen Confidence Workshops. Emphasize that these workshops are aimed to equip readers with the skills and information required to feel confident and in charge when it comes to cooking, nutrition, and weight management.

2. Virtual and In-Person choices: - Highlight the flexibility of the workshops, including both virtual and in-person choices. This enables participants to pick the format that best matches their interests and circumstances, guaranteeing accessibility for a large audience.

3. Skill-Building Sessions: - Describe the skill-building sessions implemented within the workshops. These workshops may cover a variety of culinary skills, from fundamental knife techniques and cooking procedures to meal planning, food selection, and time-saving suggestions.

4. Nutrition Education Component: - Introduce a nutrition education component inside the sessions. Provide information on the principles of nutrition, the necessity of balanced meals, and how cooking at home may help to improve eating habits and weight control.

5. Interactive culinary demos: - Include interactive culinary demos delivered by professional educators. These demos may highlight the step-by-step creation of healthful and tasty foods, enabling participants to follow along and develop their culinary talents.

6. Q&A Sessions and Troubleshooting: - Incorporate dedicated Q&A sessions to answer participants' queries and concerns. Create an open and friendly atmosphere where folks may seek help on particular culinary issues, item substitutions, or general kitchen inquiries.

7. Recipe Customization ideas: - Provide ideas on adapting dishes to fit individual tastes and dietary demands. Empower participants to make educated decisions regarding food replacements, quantity proportions, and taste variations, encouraging a feeling of creativity and agility in the kitchen.

8. Meal Planning tactics: - Include talks on successful meal-planning tactics. Guide participants on how to plan meals for the week, balance nutritional needs, and simplify the cooking process for increased efficiency and consistency.

9. making tasty and healthful meals: - Focus on making tasty and healthful meals. Explore strategies for boosting taste without depending on excessive salt or harmful substances, enabling participants to enjoy the richness of natural tastes.

10. Culinary Confidence Boosters: - Share strategies and practices to increase culinary confidence. This can include tips for overcoming typical kitchen phobias, experimenting with new ingredients, and having a positive approach toward the culinary process.

11. Progress Tracking and Celebrations: - Incorporate progress-tracking systems inside the sessions. Encourage participants to celebrate their successes, whether it's learning a new culinary technique, regularly making home-cooked meals, or attaining particular nutrition and weight control objectives.

12. Community involvement and Support: - Foster community involvement and support among workshop participants. Create a forum for sharing triumphs, swapping recipes, and offering support, developing a network of persons on a shared road toward kitchen confidence and healthy living.

By conducting culinary Confidence Workshops, the cookbook strives to bridge the gap between readers' present culinary abilities and their desires for improved cooking and eating habits. The sessions offer a friendly and instructional atmosphere where people may obtain the confidence and information required to take charge of their nutrition and weight management journey.

www.ingramcontent.com/pod-product-compliance
Lightning Source LLC
Chambersburg PA
CBHW070818260726
48660CB00005B/1892